The Simp Diet Guide for Beginners + 35 Recipes

Low FODMAP Diet: What to Do and What to Avoid

Eric P. Garvin

We want to thank you for downloading this book "IBS (Irritable Bowel Syndrome) Diet: Low FODMAP Diet, What to Do and What to Avoid + 35 Recipes."

How often do you feel a sudden cramp-like pain in your stomach and take it for granted? How often do you find yourself in awkward situations, constantly feeling the urge to use the washroom? Do you feel bloated all the time?

If you have been faced with any of these situations, you are not alone. In fact, about 48 million Americans are currently experiencing the same problem. It seems that population of our country is most affected with irritable bowel syndrome, which is caused by our lifestyle and eating habits.

This book is a sincere attempt to inform you about irritable bowel syndrome and help you to be cured of it. We don't want to overwhelm you with too much information, so the main body of our book focuses on finding solutions instead of dwelling on the problem. Besides explaining how irritable bowels can disrupt your life, we also explain how a low FODMAP diet can help you to regain your health faster. Have you never heard of a low FODMAP diet? Well, you will learn everything about it in the coming chapters.

The primary focus of this book is to provide you with lots of low FODMAP recipes. We want to help you to change your eating habits that you will never have to suffer from this condition again.

Most people do not know what is a low FODMAP diet. So it makes sense that not many chefs have come up with recipes, which are suitable for a low FODMAP diet. On the other hand, we have spent enough time. We have carefully created over 35 super-easy recipes that will help you to heal faster. In this book, we are giving you about seven recipes for each of breakfast, soup, lunch, dinner and dessert. These recipes are super-easy to follow and to make.

The goal of this book is to end your search for much-needed relief from irritable bowel syndrome. You deserve to lead a life that is free of diseases or debilitating medical conditions. This is one you can do something about. Reading this book should help you to get there. Happy reading!

Tabe of Contents

Chapter 1: What are irritable bowel syndrome (IBS) and the low FODMAP diet?

What is irritable bowel syndrome?

Irritable bowel syndrome is a medical condition, wherein the patient experiences abdominal pain, irregular bowel movements, constipation, bloating and diarrhoea. Although the exact cause of IBS is not known, some factors that can lead to an irritable bowel include eating too much junk food, lack of hydration, family medical history, and excessive stress. When the condition becomes extreme, sufferers may even pass blood through their stools. If you experience a severe symptom, go immediately to your doctor and get treatment. If IBS left untreated for a long time, it can disrupt your life and will certainly prevent you from leading a normal life.

What is a low FODMAP diet?

FODMAP is an acronym. It stands for Fermentable Oligosaccharides, Disaccharides, Monosaccharides and Polyols.

These are the names of complex molecules that are found in food, which some people find difficult to absorb. The lack of absorption of these molecules may cause the accumulation of harmful bacteria inside the tummy, eventually resulting in irritable bowels.

The low FODMAP diet helps to combat all sorts of bowel issues, Crohn's disease and other intestinal and stomach problems.

Chapter 2: Explanation of FODMAP symptoms

Meals lead to bloating

FODMAP ingredients, such as fructose, are easily absorbed through the small intestine by most people, but some people experience immense difficulty with this. When the fructose enters the large intestine, it is defined almost as a foreign body, often resulting in the proliferation of more bacteria in the gut. This situation can result in constant bloating, constipation or diarrhoea. Some people experience immense pain in their guts, which is caused by excessive gas.

This intolerance ends up, causing further problems in the body including fatigue, restlessness and lack of sleep. People, who suffer from this intolerance, often cringe at the thought of eating food as the after-effects are difficult to tolerate.

Foods, which are considered to be healthy, often aggravate the symptoms

Most people and most experts believe that healthy food equates to fruits, vegetables, legumes and whole grains. While these foods are certainly beneficial, most can be highly problematic for people, who suffer from irritable bowel. Why? Because all these foods contain higher levels of fructose, which makes it difficult for some people to digest it.

While some of these foods are lower in fructose content, others contain marginally high amounts of it. Therefore, it is important to know, which foods are in the low FODMAP category. Whole grains, for example, are considered healthy, but they are high in fructans (fructan is a polymer of fructose molecules) and must be avoided to alleviate IBS symptoms.

Discontinue lactose even, if you are not lactose intolerant

Not everyone, who suffers from FODMAP sensitivities, is lactose intolerant. Some may not have any problems with dairy products at all. Regardless, it is helpful to eliminate dairy from your daily diet, as it can contribute to your irritable bowel issues to some extent. Dairy products may be absolutely useless for you, and you may think that continuing to include dairy in your diet will not harm. But it's highly likely that you will suffer from intolerance to dairy sooner or later. It's just better to be safe.

Unable to identify the cause

Many people spend years of their life battling bloating issue without being able to determine exactly, what's causing it. We tend not to look into the issue until other symptoms arise or the bloating becomes unbearable. Lots of people resort to the Internet for self-diagnosis.

While the world of the Internet is very helpful, it is also so easy to be misled by the information, which we find there. The information, which we get from the Internet, can serve us only to some extent. It can't beat the years of experience, which a doctor brings to the table. If you experience an aggravated symptom, immediately consult your doctor. Don't wait.

When consultation with a doctor doesn't help

Your doctor may not be able to determine the cause of your irritable bowel syndrome and therefore might not give any useful piece of advice for you. What should you do in such a situation? All you can do is try to learn more about your symptoms by paying attention to what makes them worse and what reduces them.

We know one person, who thought that he was lactose intolerant because eating ice cream brought on IBS symptoms. But one day he read something about carrageenan, an ingredient, which is used in many pet foods as a thickener and stabilizer, and that it acts as a laxative on dogs and cats, who are sensitive to it.

This person knew that carrageenan is used in ice cream to keep it from developing crystals, when it is in the freezer. He had always experienced IBS symptoms after eating ice cream and had always thought that he was lactose intolerant. But he knew that ice cream has carrageenan in it to keep it from developing crystals in the freezer, so he decided to investigate that.

It turned out that the evaporated milk in his mom's corn chowder recipe and coffee cream contain carrageenan. Both of these things had been causing extreme IBS symptoms for him. He knows now that he is not lactose intolerant. He needs to watch out for carrageenan on every label.

Carrageenan is a natural product; it is made from seaweed. But it's like a poison ivy attack inside our intestines every time we eat it. The people, who are sensitive to it, experience IBS and eventually learn to stay away from it. The rest of us just continue to eat products that contain it.

Pay attention, take notes, read labels. It's not the same for everybody. For some people, lactose intolerance is the cause of their inability to eat ice cream. For others, the problem is the carrageenan in the ice cream.

This is one example of how paying attention can help you to isolate your real food enemy. For most people with IBS, it is not just one thing. You will be safe, if you stick to a low FODMAP menu all the time.

Your doctor has likely advised you to add more fibre to your diet, so you've started eating tons of fruits and vegetables without knowing about the low FODMAP food chart. This could aggravate your problem instead of alleviating it, simply because you don't know, which veggies and fruits are on the low FODMAP list.

Unfortunately, most doctors do not advise the nutritional training that could actually play an important role in your recovery.

In addition to consulting a physician, you could also consult a certified nutritionist to reduce your irritable bowel symptoms.

Frequent use of the bathroom

Most people, who suffer from an irritable bowel, often experience extreme constipation or diarrhoea. Constipation is caused by not enough water intake or not enough fibre intake. Lack of hydration leads the bowel content to dry up and causes the slow movement of bowels. Extreme constipation can make it difficult for the body to pass stools, eventually resulting in anal fissures, fistula or haemorrhoids.

On the other hand, excessive liquid, which enters your bowels, causes diarrhoea. Food material moves too quickly through the bowels and there isn't enough time for the colon to dry out, as it normally would. If diarrhoea persists for a long time, it can cause inflammation of the colon, which paves the way for even more bacteria to accumulate in the bowel.

If you feel the constant urge to empty your bowel, this is a huge indicator that something is wrong with your bowel. This symptom is enough reason for your immediate consulting with your doctor.

Chapter 3: Irritable Bowel Syndrome diagnosis

Irritable bowel syndrome is rather difficult to confirm as most people in the United States suffer from many digestive disorders due to unhealthy food habits. There are no tests that can specifically diagnose irritable bowel syndrome. It can only be diagnosed through persistent symptoms, which related to the digestive system.

Your general physician will usually ask you to pay attention to what exactly is triggering your symptoms. If there is a family history of irritable bowel problems, the doctor needs to know it. To help the doctor to make a proper analysis, he will also need to know how often symptoms occur and how quickly they go away.

Ensure that you fully co-operate with your doctor to help him to make an accurate diagnosis. The best thing you can do is to write down a list of your symptoms, their duration, and what has preceded their cessation. Bring that list to your doctor. This may save time for you and your doctor, as your doctor will be working with all of the pertinent information.

Here are the most common questions that your doctor will ask, attempting to get to the bottom of your irritable bowel issues:

➢ How frequently do you have the urge to urinate or defecate?

➢ Does emptying your bowel reduce your abdominal pain?

➢ How stressful is your daily life and does extra stress seem to aggravate the symptoms?

➢ Do your stools look different on days that you are experiencing symptoms?

➢ How painful is it for you to pass stools?

➢ Does eating a heavy meal causes your tummy to feel bloated or gassy?

➢ How much water do you drink?

➢ How often do you exercise?

➢ Do you have a past history of food allergies?

➢ Do you feel a dip in your energy level, when the symptoms show up?

➢ Have you been taking any medication for your irritable bowel issues?

➢ Have the symptoms affected your sleep?

➢ How anxious or irritable do you feel throughout the day?

After you answer your doctor's questions, you will be given an appropriate line of treatment. This could include antibiotics, changes in your daily diet, regular physical activity, as well as changes in your lifestyle. If you wish to cure your bowel issues, you must stick to the line of treatment, which is advised by your doctor. Following this treatment, you may notice improvement within a month.

Chapter 4: What is a low FODMAP diet?

FODMAP is basically sugar, which is not easily digestible and can wreak havoc on your bowel.

Fermentable

This refers to the process of the gut bacteria, breaking down carbohydrates that are not digested. Gases such as carbon dioxide, hydrogen and methane are the result. Here are some of these carbohydrates:

- Fructooligosaccarides (also called fructans)

- Oligosaccharides

- Galactooligosaccharides

- Disaccharides

- Lactose

- Monosaccharide

- Fructose

- Polyols

These include sugar polyols, such as mannitol and sorbitol.

So, now, here is a list of the foods that you should eat and the foods you should avoid to maintain a low FODMAP diet. It is impossible to list all the foods that fall on either side, but this is a comprehensive list.

Foods to avoid:

- Fruits: apples, blackberries, black prunes, cherries, mangoes, nectarines, peaches, pears, plums, watermelon.

- Veggies: artichokes, asparagus, avocados, cabbage, cauliflower, garlic, mushrooms, peas, onions.

- Legumes: all except chickpeas and lentils, which you can have in small quantities as per your digestive capacity.

- Nuts: avoid cashews and pistachios at all costs; all other nuts are fine.

- Sweeteners: artificial sweeteners, honey, corn syrup and canned fruit juice.

Foods to embrace:

- Fruits: bananas, blueberries, grapes, kiwis, lemons, oranges, passion fruits, pineapple, pumpkin, strawberries, rhubarb.

- Veggies: bell peppers, broccoli, carrots, cucumber, eggplant, ginger, lettuce, potatoes, sweet potatoes, tomatoes, zucchini.

- Substitutes for onions and garlic: if a recipe asks for onions, use leeks or scallions instead. If a recipe asks for garlic, use shallots instead. Shallots taste like a combination of onions and garlic. Onion greens are okay, cooked or not. Onion bulbs you should only eat raw. Cooking activates the bad chemicals. It is the same with garlic. Cooking activates the bad chemicals in garlic, but you can absolutely use minced garlic in your tzatziki. To sum up, here are the substitutes for onions and garlic: leek, chives, scallions, shallots and onion greens. Experiment with them!

- Grains and starches: amaranth, arrowroot, buckwheat, maize (corn), millet, oats, quinoa, rice, tapioca.

- Sweeteners: brown sugar, cane sugar, icing sugar, maple syrup, palm sugar, rice syrup.

Chapter 5: Three common mistakes that people make, while attempting a low FODMAP diet

What should you do, if your symptoms are not alleviated by your new low FODMAP diet? Are your hopes fading? Well, there are three common mistakes you might make:

1. Eating too much at one sitting

Being on a low FODMAP diet doesn't mean that it is okay to overeat. While you may get excited about how light you feel, when you've embarked on a low FODMAP diet, eating too much at one sitting can put pressure on your bowel. This does not mean that you must starve or skip meals. The key to getting it right is maintaining a balance. Eat smaller meals more frequently to make it easier for your gut to break down the food.

Keep your body hydrated by drinking enough water during the day, as it is vital for your recovery. What is more important, you need to know, when to drink water. Drink enough liquid two hours before eating and again an hour after meals. By keeping your liquid intake from interfering with the digestive process, your body can digest your food without much effort.

2. Eating processed foods

At all costs, stay away from all processed foods. Always check the label and watch out for ingredients that you have never heard of. If you see one single ingredient on the list that you don't recognize, don't even think of buying it. Before you start on your low FODMAP diet, ensure that your kitchen is free of such processed foods. Throw away all packaged items and never buy them again. Does this seem like an extreme step to you? Do it anyway, because packaged foods are extremely toxic and will do your body a lot of harm in the long run.

Does this mean that we must throw away packages of rice and flour too? No, you don't need to throw away packages that contain one single ingredient such as rice, flour or rice flour, because they only contain that one ingredient and nothing else. The packages, which you need to eliminate, are the ones that include complex ingredients, completely unfamiliar to you.

Get rid of packaged foods such as ready-to-make food packets, packaged meats and sauces right away.

3. Holding on for too long

You are at a party or a conference and fighting your urge to use the washroom to avoid embarrassment. Think for a minute. Is it really worth it? Suppressing your urge to empty your bowel only puts more pressure on your bowel. In such circumstances, do not hesitate to use the washroom as many times as you want.

Firstly, not everyone is interested in observing, how many times you are using the washroom. Secondly, even if someone does, you need to prioritize your health over such trivial matters and stop caring about what others think. If you keep fighting these urges, your recovery will just take longer. Decide what you want: a fast recovery or avoiding embarrassment. Take your pick.

Chapter 6: Tips for reducing IBS symptoms naturally

Peppermint oil

Many people find relief through peppermint oil. Peppermint oil supplements, which are taken twice daily between meals, can reduce flatulence and IBS-related pain. Peppermint tea is also widely used to enhance digestion and relieve chronic constipation. Before using peppermint oil or peppermint tea, consult a doctor. Peppermint can exacerbate conditions, such as acid reflux.

Lots of water

Experts advise drinking two to three litres of water a day to maintain a healthy digestive tract. If you are suffering from irritable bowel syndrome, your water intake should be at least three litres each and every day. As it is explained above, it is equally vital that you know, when to drink water. Do not flood your digestive system with water immediately before or after eating food, as it slows down the digestion process. Water keeps you hydrated during the day and also ensures that your stools are loosened up, so they don't put too much pressure on the bowel.

Reduce stress

Stress is hugely responsible for disturbances in our lives, both mental and physical. A stress-free life is important in keeping bowel irritability at bay. Raised anxiety levels, which are caused by daily stress, can aggravate any such underlying problems.

If your life is stressful, try participating in activities, such as yoga or meditation to help you to maintain a peaceful state of mind. Also, treat yourself with spas, herbal teas and anything else that relaxes you.

Be active

If your lifestyle has been sedentary, it is now time to move your butt. Make physical exercise a part of your daily routine. If your job requires you to sit in one position for long periods of time, get up and move around for a few minutes each hour. Just keep yourself moving. When you exercise, your body automatically relieves itself of stress and floods your brain with happy endorphins. When you are truly happy in life, your body can cure itself faster than, if you are not happy.

Herbal teas for alleviating IBS symptoms

The studies have shown that herbal teas have a calming effect on your body as a whole and they also reduce IBS symptoms. Chamomile and peppermint tea especially have become hugely popular among people suffering from irritable bowel syndrome. Bring a cup of water to a boil. Add a teaspoon of chamomile tea and let it seep for 10-15 minutes to get maximum flavour and maximum soothing.

Conclusion

Thank you again for buying this book. Irritable bowel syndrome is not a condition to be taken lightly. Initially, the bloating, cramps and frequent need to use the bathroom may merely be inconvenient, but they can turn your life upside down in no time. We hope that after reading this book you will not ignore this condition and you will take serious steps towards treating it. You will have to make some lifestyle changes and tweak your eating habits to ensure it doesn't reappear.

If your doctor advises you to adopt a low FODMAP diet, you don't have waste your valuable time looking all over the Internet to find recipes, which you can use. Feel free to give our recipes your own twist, but remember to adhere to the low FODMAP diet chart by adding veggies and fruits of your choice.

We hope that this comprehensive guide will make your journey easier and enjoyable at the same time.

Chapter 7: Low FODMAP Soups

1. Carrot, Ginger, and Coconut Soup

Serves: 4

Ingredients

- 8 medium carrots
- 4 parsnips
- 8 cups of vegetable stock
- 2 teaspoons of salt
- 1 teaspoon of ground pepper
- 1 tablespoon of minced ginger
- 1 teaspoon of turmeric
- 1 tablespoon of paprika
- 1 cup of thick coconut milk
- 1 tablespoon of apple cider vinegar
- 2 tablespoons of sunflower seeds for garnish

Method

1. Wash the carrots and parsnips, peel and chop them into small chunks. Set aside.

2. Pour the vegetable broth into a large saucepan.

3.   Add salt and pepper to taste and bring the broth to a boil.

4.   Slide in the chopped veggies and add the minced ginger, paprika and turmeric. Simmer for about 20 minutes until the veggies are tender.

5.   Allow the mixture to cool and drain off the stock. Set the stock aside.

6.   Using a blender, mix the veggies until you have a lump-free smooth paste.

7.   Transfer this paste back into the saucepan and pour the stock back in with it.

8.   Add coconut milk and apple cider vinegar. Stir, using a large wooden spoon.

9.   Simmer for about 5 minutes until it thickens slightly.

10.   Garnish with sunflower seeds and serve.

2. Low FODMAP Minestrone Soup

Serves: 4-5

Ingredients

- 3 medium slices of uncured bacon

- 2 large carrots, chopped or diced

- 1 large potato, chopped or diced

- 1 cup of chopped leek (or scallions)

- 1 stalk celery, chopped or diced

- 1 tablespoon of olive oil

- 2 cup of crushed tomatoes

- 1 teaspoon of salt

- 1 teaspoon of ground pepper

- 2 tablespoons of lemon juice

- 3 cups of vegetable stock

- ¾ cup of gluten-free pasta

- 1 cup of baby spinach, roughly chopped

- fresh basil leaves for garnish

- 1 tablespoon of grated parmesan cheese for garnish

Method

1.   Fry the uncured bacon slices and chop into chunks.

2.   Prepare the carrots, potato, leek and celery.

3.   Heat a large saucepan over medium heat and add olive oil.

4.   Sauté the carrots, potato, leek, celery and bacon bits. Continue sautéing for 3-4 minutes until the veggies are tender.

5.   Add crushed tomatoes, salt, pepper and lemon juice. Cook for 3 more minutes.

6.   Slowly pour the vegetable stock into the pan and mix the ingredients well.

7.   Slide in the pasta and the spinach and stir well.

8.   Simmer the soup for about 10 minutes until all ingredients are cooked.

9.   Transfer into soup bowls and add some grated cheese on top.

10.   Garnish with fresh parsley.

11.   Serve hot.

3. Easy Ratatouille

Serves: 4

Ingredients

- 3 tablespoons of extra virgin olive oil, divided
- 1 large egg plant, sliced
- 2 small zucchinis, peeled and chopped
- ½ cup of thin green beans
- 1 large red bell pepper, sliced
- 2 cups of diced ripe tomatoes
- 1 teaspoon of red chili flakes
- 1 teaspoon of salt
- 1 teaspoon of cayenne pepper
- 1 tablespoon of mixed dried herbs
- ¼ cup of olives, roughly chopped
- fresh basil leaves, chopped, for garnish

Method

1. Heat one tablespoon of extra virgin olive oil in a flat saucepan over medium heat.

2. Add the eggplant slices to it and fry them on both sides until they turn golden brown. Transfer them to a bowl.

3.   Add 2 tablespoons of extra virgin olive oil to the same saucepan and keep it cooking over medium heat.

4.   Add the zucchini, green beans and bell pepper. Cook for 3-4 minutes until veggies are thoroughly tender.

5.   Throw in the diced tomatoes. Cook for another 5-6 minutes until they are soft.

6.   Stir in the fried eggplant slices, red chili flakes, salt, cayenne pepper and dried herbs. Cover the pan with a lid.

7.   Continue cooking for 20 to 25 minutes until the sauce has completely thickened.

8.   Now stir in the chopped olives.

9.   Transfer the mixture into soup bowls.

10.   Garnish with fresh basil leaves.

11.   Serve hot.

4. Potato and Spinach Soup

Serves: 4

Ingredients

- cooking spray

- 8 slices of uncured bacon

- 5 large potatoes

- 1 tablespoon of vegetable oil

- 1 tablespoon of minced ginger

- 1 stalk celery, chopped

- 1 red chilli, slit

- 1 cup of baby spinach

- 1 cup of green beans

- 1 ¼ teaspoon of salt

- 1 teaspoon of ground black pepper

- 1 teaspoon of cumin powder

- 1 teaspoon of paprika

- ½ cup of thick tomato puree

- 4 cups of chicken stock

- fresh mint leaves and chives, finely chopped, for garnish

Method

1.   Spray a small saucepan with cooking oil and heat it over medium heat.

2.   Sauté the uncured bacon slices for 2 to 3 minutes on each side. Chop them into chunks or bits and set aside.

3.   Wash and peel the potatoes, cut into small chunks.

4.   Heat a tablespoon of vegetable oil in a large saucepan over medium heat.

5.   Add the minced ginger, chopped celery, red chilli and fry for 2 to 3 minutes.

6.   Add the potato chunks to the pan and fry for 3 minutes until they are slightly browned.

7.   Throw in the baby spinach and green beans. Add salt, pepper, cumin and paprika. Cook for 3 more minutes.

8.   Add the tomato puree and simmer for 5 minutes.

9.   Slowly pour the chicken stock into the pan. Simmer the soup for 15 minutes until all the ingredients are cooked.

10.   Once the mixture cools down, use a blender to mix until you have a smooth lump-free soup.

11.   Transfer this soup back to the pan and add the uncured bacon bits.

12.   Simmer again for 5 more minutes.

13. Garnish with chopped mint leaves and chives.

14. Serve hot.

5. Roasted Vegetable Soup

Serves: 4

Ingredients

- 1 large red bell pepper
- 1 large yellow bell pepper
- 2 cups of plum tomatoes, diced
- 1 medium eggplant, sliced
- 1 large celery, chopped
- 2 tablespoons of olive oil
- 2 tablespoons of brown sugar
- 1 tablespoon of balsamic vinegar
- 1 teaspoon of dried thyme
- 1 teaspoon of dried oregano
- 1 teaspoon of salt
- 5 cups of vegetable stock
- 1 teaspoon of ground black pepper
- 2 tablespoons of lime juice
- chopped parsley for garnish

Method

1. Preheat the oven to 390 degrees F (200 C).

2.   Mix the red bell pepper, yellow bell pepper, tomatoes, eggplant and celery and spread them out on a prepared baking sheet.

3.   Toss together in a bowl the olive oil, sugar, balsamic vinegar, thyme, oregano and salt.

4.   Pour this mixture over the vegetables and roast them in the oven for about 35 minutes until they are completely golden brown.

5.   Add the vegetable stock to a large pot and bring it to a boil. Add the roasted vegetables to the stock. Simmer for about 10 minutes until the stock reduces.

6.   Once it cools down, use a blender to blend until a smooth paste is obtained.

7.   Transfer the soup back to the pan, add pepper and lime juice. Stir well.

8.   Garnish with chopped parsley and serve.

6. Gluten Free Seafood Chowder

Serves: 4

Ingredients

For the fish stock

- 2 medium potatoes, diced
- 2 medium carrots, diced
- 3 shallots, diced
- 1 medium leek, diced
- 1 teaspoon of dried thyme
- 1 teaspoon of dried oregano
- 1 teaspoon of salt
- 1 teaspoon of ground black pepper
- 2 bay leaves
- 3 slices of uncured bacon
- 2 cups of white water fish
- 1 cup of prawn heads and shells
- 2 cups of white wine
- 1 tablespoon of olive oil
- 6-7 cups of water

For the chowder

- 12 medium prawns

- 1 cup of white flesh fish

- ½ teaspoon of salt

- 1 teaspoon of turmeric

- A handful of clams

- ½ cup of cream (optional)

- ½ teaspoon of ground pepper

- 1 tablespoon of potato starch

- chopped parsley for garnish

Method

1. Add all the ingredients for the fish stock to a large pot. Bring it to a boil.

2. Strain off the fish stock, transfer it to a saucepan and bring it to a boil again. Throw away the rest of the stuff that was used to make the fish stock.

3. Lower the heat. Add prawns, fish, salt and turmeric. Stir.

4. Add the clams and let the mixture to simmer for 7-8 minutes.

5. Add some cream (optional), followed by ground pepper. Mix together well.

6. Stir in the potato starch. Simmer for 2 to 3 minutes until the mixture thickens.

7. Garnish with chopped parsley.

8. Serve hot.

7. Quinoa and Tomato Soup

Serves: 4

Ingredients

- 6 medium carrots
- 2 tablespoons of olive oil
- 3 tablespoons of roasted cumin powder
- 1 tablespoon of smoked paprika
- 8 medium tomatoes, diced
- 2 cup of rainbow Swiss chard, roughly chopped
- 1 small eggplant, chopped
- 2 large red bell peppers, chopped
- ¼ cup of gluten-free soy sauce
- ½ cup of chopped leek greens
- ½ cup of thick tomato paste
- 1 ½ teaspoon of salt
- 1 teaspoon of cayenne pepper
- 1 tablespoon of maple syrup
- 8 cups of vegetable stock
- 1 cup of sprouted quinoa
- Some chopped coriander for garnish

Method

1.　Wash and peel the carrots. Chop into small chunks or slices.

2.　Heat some olive oil in a large saucepan over medium heat.

3.　Add the carrots along with the cumin and paprika. Sauté 3 to 4 minutes until the carrots are tender.

4.　Meanwhile, bring some water to a boil in a large pot. Add the tomatoes and Swiss chard. Let it keep boiling for about 2 minutes and then drain the excess water. Add the tomatoes and Swiss chard to a blender and blend until a smooth paste is obtained.

5.　Pour this mixture into the saucepan with the carrots. Add the chopped eggplant and bell peppers. Cover and cook for 3 minutes on high temperature.

6.　Add the soy sauce, leek greens, tomato paste, salt, cayenne pepper and maple syrup. Mix well.

7.　Pour the vegetable broth slowly into the mixture, stirring continuously.

8.　Add the quinoa and cover the pan with a lid.

9.　Cook for about 35 minutes until all ingredients are completely cooked.

10.　Transfer to soup bowls, garnish with chopped coriander.

11.　Serve hot.

Chapter 8: IBS Breakfast Recipes

1. Banana Nut Bread

Serves: around 16 slices

Ingredients

- 2 large ripe bananas, peeled
- 2 cups of almond flour
- ¼ teaspoon of salt
- ½ teaspoon of baking powder
- 1 teaspoon of baking soda
- 1/3 cup of brown sugar
- ½ teaspoon of ground cinnamon
- 3 large egg-whites
- ½ cup of almond milk
- 1 teaspoon of vanilla extract
- 1/3 cup of coconut oil
- ½ cup of chopped almonds and walnuts for topping

Method

1. Preheat the oven to 300 degrees F (150 C).

2.   Using your hands, mash the bananas in a bowl. Set aside.

3.   In another bowl, combine the almond flour with salt, baking powder, baking soda, brown sugar and cinnamon. Mix well.

4.   Add the egg-whites to another bowl and whisk them until they are frothy. You can use a hand blender.

5.   Slide in the mashed bananas, almond milk, vanilla extract, coconut oil. Mix.

6.   Pour this mixture into the flour mixture and mix well, using a large spoon.

7.   Transfer the batter to a prepared baking pan and top it up with chopped almonds and walnuts.

8.   Cover with foil and bake for 55 minutes.

9.   Allow the bread to cool on a rack for 15 minutes.

10.   Slice and serve. You can also store it in an airtight container for up to 7 days.

2. Scrambled Eggs & Sourdough Toast

Serves: 1

Ingredients

- olive oil for the frying pan

- 2 eggs

- a splash of milk or almond milk

- dash of salt

- dash of ground black pepper

- 1 tablespoon of grated cheese

- traditional sourdough bread (containing only flour, water, salt and no extra yeast)

- ground paprika for garnish

Method

1. In a bowl whisk the eggs with a splash of milk.

2. Whisk in the salt and pepper.

3. Fold in the grated cheese.

4. Pour into a skillet with olive oil, which is set over medium heat.

5. Stir the eggs a bit as they set.

6. Put some bread in the toaster.

7. Put the eggs on the toast and sprinkle with paprika.

8. Eat.

3. Strawberries and Almond Milk Oatmeal

Serves: 4

Ingredients

- ½ cup of fresh ripe strawberries

- 3 cups of almond milk

- 2 tablespoons of brown sugar

- 1 ½ cup of gluten oats

- 1 teaspoon of vanilla extract

- ¼ teaspoon of ground cardamom

- ⅛ teaspoon of salt

- Some chopped almonds and walnuts

Method

1. Wash the strawberries and pat them dry. Chop them roughly and set them aside.

2. Add the milk to a large pot and bring it to a boil.

3. Lower the heat and sprinkle the brown sugar into the milk. Stir until it dissolves.

4. Slide in the oats along with vanilla extract, cardamom powder and salt. Stir well with a large wooden spoon.

5.   Simmer for 5-6 minutes.

6.   Add the strawberries and cover the pot with a lid.

7.   Cook on medium heat for about 5-6 minutes more. Remove from heat and let sit for 5 more minutes before removing the lid.

8.   Heat a saucepan and add some chopped almonds and walnuts to it. Slightly toast them on all sides for 2-3 minutes.

9.   Sprinkle them on top of the oats and serve.

4. Low-Fat Apple Pumpkin Spice Bread

Serves: about 16 slices

Ingredients

- 2 cups of almond flour
- ¼ teaspoon of salt
- ½ cup of brown sugar
- 1 tablespoon of allspice powder
- ½ teaspoon of ground cinnamon
- ½ teaspoon of baking powder
- 1 teaspoon of baking soda
- 4 egg-whites
- ¼ cup of canola oil
- ¼ teaspoon of minced ginger
- 1 large cup of ripe pumpkin slices
- ½ teaspoon of vanilla extract
- 1 medium apple

Method

1. Preheat the oven to 350 degrees F (180 C).

2.   In a bowl, combine the almond flour with salt, brown sugar, allspice powder, cinnamon, baking powder, baking soda. Mix well, using a spoon.

3.   Add the egg-whites to another bowl and whisk them, using a blender until they are frothy.

4.   Use a blender to make a smooth puree out of the egg-whites, canola oil, ginger, pumpkin slices and vanilla extract.

5.   Carefully mix the egg-white mixture into the almond flour mixture to make a batter.

6.   Pour the batter into a prepared baking pan.

7.   Wash and peel the apple. Using a sharp knife, cut it into thin slices.

8.   Lay these apple slices on top of the batter in the pan.

9.   Cover the pan with foil and bake for 50 minutes.

10.   Allow the bread to cool on the rack for 15 minutes.

11.   Slice and serve. You can also store it in an airtight container for up to 7 days.

5. Blueberry and Coconut Muffins

Serves: 12 muffins

Ingredients

- ½ cup of fresh blueberries
- 1 cup of gluten-free flour
- ½ teaspoon of baking soda
- ⅛ teaspoon of salt
- ¼ teaspoon of ground cinnamon
- 2 egg-whites
- ½ teaspoon of vanilla extract
- 4 tablespoons of olive oil
- ¼ cup of brown sugar
- ¼ cup of coconut milk
- 5 tablespoons of desiccated coconut
- 7-8 chopped almonds

Method

1. Preheat the oven to 350 degrees F (180 C).

2. Wash the blueberries and pat them dry, using a paper towel. Chop them up roughly, using a sharp kitchen knife. Set aside.

3.   In a bowl, combine the flour, baking soda, salt and cinnamon. Mix well.

4.   In another bowl, whisk the egg-whites slightly with a blender.

5.   Add to the egg-whites: the vanilla extract, butter, sugar and coconut milk. Whisk once again.

6.   Add the flour mixture to the egg-white mixture bowl. Mix thoroughly. You can give the mixture a slight whisk, using a blender. Ensure there are no lumps.

7.   Gently fold in the desiccated coconut and the chopped blueberries.

8.   Pour the mixture into silicon muffin molds. Top them with chopped almonds.

9.   Bake for about 20 minutes.

10.   Allow to cool for 5 minutes.

11.   Sprinkle more desiccated coconut on top and serve.

6. Quinoa and Chicken Salad

Serves: 4

Ingredients

- 1 small cup of baby spinach

- 2 tablespoons of apple cider vinegar

- 2 ½ cups of water

- 1 cup of quinoa

- 2 teaspoons of minced ginger

- 1 small green bell pepper, diced

- 1 stalk of celery, chopped

- ½ teaspoon of salt

- ½ teaspoon of ground pepper

- 1 large chicken breast

- 4 tablespoons of extra virgin olive oil

- chopped coriander for garnish

Method

1.   Roughly chop the baby spinach and put it in a bowl. Toss well with apple cider vinegar. Set aside.

2.   Meanwhile, bring the water to a boil in a large pot.

3.   Add the quinoa to the pot and cover with a lid. Cook for 10 minutes, covered. Drain the excess water once done. Set aside in a large bowl.

4.   To the bowl of quinoa add the minced ginger, bell pepper, celery, salt and ground pepper. Mix well, using a spoon.

5.   Add the spinach and toss.

6.   Clean the chicken and pat it dry, using paper towels. Season with salt and pepper.

7.   Heat a pan over medium heat.

8.   Using olive oil, sauté the chicken breast on all sides for 4-5 minutes, until it is golden brown.

9.   Shred the chicken, using a kitchen knife. Add it to the bowl with the quinoa mixture.

10.   Garnish with chopped coriander and serve.

7. Gluten Free Cinnamon Buckwheat Pancakes

Serves: around 6

Ingredients

- 1 cup of buckwheat flour
- ¼ teaspoon of salt
- 1 teaspoon of baking powder
- 1 teaspoon of baking soda
- 2 tablespoons of palm sugar
- ½ teaspoon of ground cinnamon
- 1 large organic egg
- ½ teaspoon of vanilla extract
- 1 cup of coconut milk
- Some coconut oil for the pan
- 2 tablespoons of honey for topping
- 7-8 strawberries, chopped, for topping

Method

1.   In a bowl, combine the buckwheat flour with the salt, baking powder, baking soda, palm sugar and ground cinnamon. Mix with a spoon.

2.   Crack an egg into another bowl. Add the vanilla extract and coconut milk. Whisk with a blender.

3.   Slowly add the flour mixture to the egg bowl and whisk all the ingredients to form a smooth batter.

4.   Heat some coconut oil in a skillet or griddle over medium heat.

5.   Slowly pour a dollop of batter on the skillet and spread it evenly using a spatula.

6.   Cook for about 2-3 minutes until you see a bubble texture on the top.

7.   Flip the pancake and cook for another 2 minutes until it turns slightly brown.

8.   Repeat this step with the remaining pancake batter and make more pancakes.

9.   Drizzle honey and sprinkle strawberries on top and serve.

Chapter 9: Low FODMAP Lunch Recipes

1. Cilantro Ginger Chicken Meatballs

Serves: 4

Ingredients

- 1 pound of chicken breast

- ¾ teaspoon of salt

- ¾ teaspoon of ground black pepper

- half a green chilli, finely chopped

- 1 tablespoon of minced ginger

- 1 teaspoon of fish sauce

- 1 tablespoon of soy sauce

- 1 small leek (or several scallions), chopped

- chopped cilantro

- 1 egg-white

- peanut coconut, drizzle for garnish

Method

1. Preheat the oven to 350 degrees F (180 C).

2.   Wash the chicken breast and pat dry, using paper towels.

3.   Heat a pan over medium heat and add the chicken breast.

4.   Cook for a couple of minutes on all sides until it is slightly brown.

5.   Remove the chicken from the heat and shred, using a kitchen knife.

6.   Add the shredded chicken to a bowl along with the salt, pepper, green chilli, minced ginger, fish sauce, soy sauce, leek and cilantro. Mix well by using your hands.

7.   Crack an egg-white into the chicken mixture and mix again.

8.   Make small meatballs out of the mixture using your hands.

9.   Place them on a prepared baking tray.

10.   Bake for 20 minutes until they are brown.

11.   Garnish with coconut peanut sauce and serve.

2. Chicken and Sweet Potato Risotto

Serves: 4

Ingredients

For the chicken stock

- 4 cups of water

- 1 carrot, chopped

- 4 celery stalks, chopped

- 1 small leek (or several scallions or two shallots), sliced

For the risotto

- 2 medium chicken breast fillets

- 1 large sweet potato, peeled

- 1 teaspoon of salt

- 1 teaspoon of vegetable oil

- 1 cup of risotto rice

- 2 shallots, finely chopped

- ½ teaspoon of dried rosemary

- ½ teaspoon of dried oregano

- 1 teaspoon of ground black pepper

- ½ cup of chives, chopped, for garnish

Method

1.   Add all the ingredients for the stock to a large pot.

2.   Wash and pat dry the chicken. Chop it into chunks using a sharp kitchen knife.

3.   Add the chicken chunks to the pot and bring the stock to a boil.

4.   Simmer for about 20 minutes.

5.   Remove the chicken chunks to another bowl and strain off the stock.

6.   Add the sweet potato and add the slices to a prepared pan over medium heat.

7.   Fry the sweet potato slices on all sides until they are golden brown.

8.   Put the chicken stock in a pot, add the salt and bring it to a boil.

9.   Add the vegetable oil, risotto rice, chopped leek, rosemary, oregano and ground pepper. Stir.

10.   Add the fried potatoes and chicken chunks. Cover with a lid.

11.   Cook for 20 minutes.

12.   Garnish with chopped chives and serve.

3. Rice Noodles with Pork and Shrimp

Serves: 4

Ingredients

- 1 cup of rice noodles

- ½ pound of pork loin

- 1 tablespoon of olive oil

- 1 tablespoon of minced shallot

- 1 tablespoon of minced ginger

- 3 medium shallots, sliced

- 1 roasted red bell pepper, sliced

- 2 tablespoons of soy sauce

- 1 tablespoon of sugar

- 1 cup of bean sprouts

- 2 cups of chicken stock

- ¾ teaspoon of salt

- chopped cilantro for garnish

Method

1.   Boil some water in a large pot and slide the rice noodles into it. Cook for 4-5 minutes and remove from the heat. Drain the excess water and set aside.

2.   Wash and pat dry the pork loin using paper towels.

3.   Heat some olive oil in a large skillet over medium heat.

4.   Add the pork loin and cook for 2 to 3 minutes on all sides until it is slightly tender.

5.   Remove the pork from the heat and slice it into small chunks using a sharp knife.

6.   Heat about one tablespoon of olive oil in the same skillet.

7.   Add the minced shallot, ginger and shallots. Sauté for a couple of minutes until the shallots start releasing water.

8.   Throw in the roasted bell pepper slices, soy sauce, sugar, bean sprouts. Cook for 3 minutes.

9.   Add the chicken stock.

10.   Slide in the pork chunks and add the salt. Cook for 5-6 minutes, covered. Ensure that all the liquid is absorbed.

11.   Add in the rice noodles and toss all the ingredients. Keep cooking for a couple of minutes and then remove from heat.

12.   Garnish with chopped cilantro and serve.

4. Bacon Cheeseburger

Serves: 4

Ingredients

- 5-6 uncured bacon slices
- 1 pound of ground beef
- 1 teaspoon of salt
- 1 teaspoon of minced shallot
- ½ green chilli, finely chopped
- ½ teaspoon of cayenne pepper
- 1 teaspoon of dried oregano
- 1 teaspoon of dried basil
- ¼ cup of chopped chives
- 1 teaspoon of olive oil
- 4 large whole wheat hamburger buns
- ½ cup of shredded Parmesan cheese for garnish
- chopped coriander for garnish
- fresh strawberries and toothpicks for garnish

Method

1.   Heat a pan over medium heat.

2.   Add the uncured bacon slices to the pan and sauté for a couple of minutes on both sides. Chop up the uncured bacon slices.

3.   Put the uncured chopped bacon slices in a bowl along with the ground beef, salt, shallots, green chilli, pepper, oregano, basil and chives. Mix well using your hands.

4.   Make 4 large patties out of the ground beef mixture.

5.   Heat olive oil in a pan over medium heat.

6.   Add the burger patties to the pan and fry them for 3-4 minutes on each side until they have a golden brown crust.

7.   Slice the burger buns.

8.   Place the beef patties on the buns, garnish with Parmesan cheese and coriander and secure with a toothpick.

9.   Tuck in some fresh strawberries on the top of the toothpicks and serve.

5. Egg Shakshuka

Serves: 4

Ingredients

- 1 medium red bell pepper
- 1 tablespoon of olive oil
- 1 tablespoon of minced shallot
- ¼ cup of leek, chopped
- 2 cups of roughly chopped baby spinach
- 2 cups of crushed cherry tomatoes
- 1 teaspoon of salt
- ½ teaspoon of cayenne pepper
- 1 teaspoon of paprika
- 1 teaspoon of red chili flakes
- 1 teaspoon of ground cumin
- 1 cup of chicken stock
- 1 tablespoon of corn flour
- 4 egg-whites
- 8 slices of whole wheat bread

Method

1. Roast the red bell pepper over medium heat. Remove the skin and cut the pepper into thin strips.

2. Heat the olive oil in a large saucepan over medium heat.

3. Add the minced shallots and chopped leek. Sauté for a couple of minutes until the veggies start to become tender.

4. Throw in the roasted capsicum along with the chopped baby spinach. Cook for 2-3 minutes more.

5. Add the crushed tomatoes and cook for 2-3 minutes until it begins to thicken.

6. Sprinkle on the salt, pepper, paprika, red chilli flakes and cumin. Stir.

7. Pour in the chicken stock and mix all ingredients well.

8. Add a spoonful of water to the tablespoon of corn flour and mix well.

9. Add the corn flour mixture to the pan. Simmer for 4 minutes until the tomato mixture thickens.

10. Crack the egg-whites over the thickened tomato mixture and cover with a lid.

11. Cook over low heat for 10-12 minutes.

12. Serve with slices of whole-wheat bread.

6. Slow Cooker Chicken and Wild Rice

Serves: 4 to 5

Ingredients

- 1 pound of chicken breasts, skinless
- 2 tablespoons of olive oil
- 1 ½ teaspoon of salt
- 1 teaspoon of ground black pepper
- 1 tablespoon of dairy-free butter
- 1 bay leaf
- 4 medium carrots, peeled and finely chopped
- 1 large zucchini, finely chopped
- 3 cups of chicken broth
- 1 small cup of wild rice
- 1 teaspoon of dried thyme
- 2 tablespoons of lemon juice
- 2 egg yolks
- chopped parsley for garnish

Method

1. Trim the excess fat off the chicken breast.

2.   Season the chicken breast with lots of salt and pepper.

3.   Heat a pan over medium heat and add the olive oil and chicken breast. Cook chicken for 4 minutes on each side until it is golden brown. Slice it into small chunks.

4.   Melt some dairy-free butter in a slow cooker over medium heat.

5.   Add bay leaf, chopped carrots and zucchini. Sauté until the veggies are tender.

6.   Slowly pour the chicken broth into the cooker and stir all the ingredients continuously.

7.   Let the mixture simmer for 5 minutes.

8.   Add the wild rice and thyme. Sprinkle the lemon juice on top.

9.   Fold the egg yolks into the rice.

10.   Cover with a lid and cook for 4 hours on high heat.

11.   Garnish with some chopped parsley and serve.

7. Sweet and Sour Chicken with Cumin Rice

Serves: 4 to 5

Ingredients

For the chicken

- 4 tablespoons of brown sugar

- 4 tablespoons of apple cider vinegar

- 2 tablespoons of gluten-free soy sauce

- ¼ cup of chicken stock

- 1 pound of chicken breasts

- 1 egg-white

- ½ cup of cornstarch

- 4 tablespoons of coconut oil

- 1 cup of pineapple chunks

- 1 large bell pepper, sliced

- 1 teaspoon of ground black pepper

- 2 to 3 shallots, thinly sliced

- 1 teaspoon of salt

For the cumin rice

- 1 cup of water

- 1 tablespoon of cumin

- few drops of oil

- ¼ teaspoon of salt

- 1 cup of long grain rice

- chopped coriander for garnish

Method

1. Combine the brown sugar with the apple cider vinegar, soy sauce and chicken stock. Mix well.

2. Pour this mixture into a saucepan and bring to a boil over medium heat. Simmer for 5 minutes and remove from heat.

3. Wash the chicken and pat dry. Cut into small chunks.

4. Whisk the egg-white and pour it over the chicken. Add these chicken chunks to a ziplock bag along with the cornstarch and shake well to coat them.

5. Drizzle some oil on a large pan and heat over medium heat.

6. Add the coated chicken chunks to the pan and cook for 2 to 3 minutes on each side until it is crispy.

7. Add the pineapple chunks and sliced bell pepper. Sauté for a couple of minutes more.

8. Throw in the ground black pepper, shallots and salt. Sauté for a few more minutes.

9. Add the chicken stock mixture to the pan. Simmer until the mixture thickens.

10. In the meantime, boil about one cup of water in a large pot.

11. Add the cumin, a few drops of oil, the salt and then the rice. Cover and cook for 7-8 minutes. Transfer the rice mixture to a large plate.

12. Pour the chicken mixture on top.

13. Garnish with chopped coriander and serve.

Chapter 10: Low FODMAP Desserts

1. Dark Chocolate and Raspberry Brownies

Serves: 10 pieces

Ingredients

- 1 cup of dairy-free butter
- 1 cup of dark chocolate
- 1 cup of brown sugar
- 4 egg-whites
- 1 cup of all-purpose flour
- 4 tablespoons of dark cocoa powder
- 1 tablespoon of xanthan gum
- ¾ cup of raspberries
- chopped walnuts for topping

Method

1. Preheat oven to 350 degrees F (180 C).
2. Bring a large pot of water to a boil.
3. Place a large microwave bowl over the pot.

4.   Add dairy-free butter, chocolate and brown sugar to the bowl. Keep stirring until all the ingredients melt.

5.   Once the mixture is smooth, remove it from the heat and add the egg-whites. Whisk well by using a hand blender.

6.   In another bowl, combine the flour, cocoa powder and xanthan gum. Mix well.

7.   Slowly pour the flour mixture into the chocolate mixture and mix well using a spoon. Make sure there are no lumps.

8.   Lightly fold in the raspberries and pour the mixture into a prepared baking tray. Sprinkle chopped walnuts on top.

9.   Bake the brownies for about 30 minutes.

10.   Allow them to cool for 15 minutes before cutting.

11.   Serve warm.

2. Blueberry Crumble Slice

Serves: 10 slices

Ingredients

For the base

- 2 ½ cups of self-rising flour
- ¼ teaspoon of salt
- ½ teaspoon of ground cinnamon
- ¾ cup of white sugar
- 1 cup of dairy-free butter
- 1 egg-white

For the filling

- 2 1/2 cups of blueberries
- 3 teaspoons of cornflour
- ¼ cup of white sugar

Method

1.   Preheat the oven to 350 degrees F (180 C).

2.   Prepare a medium-sized baking sheet or tray with some dairy-free butter and set aside.

3.   In a bowl, combine the self-rising flour with the salt, cinnamon powder and ¾ cup of sugar. Mix well using your hands. The mixture should be slightly crumbly.

4.   Melt the dairy-free butter and pour that into the flour mixture.

5.   Crack an egg into the bowl and use your hands to knead the mixture into a firm dough.

6.   Take half of the dough and spread it evenly at the bottom of the pan.

7.   Add the blueberries as the next layer.

8.   In a small bowl, combine the corn flour with the ¼ cup of sugar and sprinkle that on top of the blueberries.

9.   Crumble the second half of the dough over the blueberries.

10.   Bake for 30 minutes until the crust is nice and golden.

11.   Cool for 15 minutes.

12.   Slice and serve.

3. Carrot and Chocolate Bundtlets

Serves: 4

Ingredients

- ¼ cup of almond milk

- 2 tablespoons of virgin coconut oil

- 1 medium carrot, pureed

- ¼ cup of brown sugar

- 1 ½ tablespoon of cocoa powder

- ½ cup of rice flour

- 1 teaspoon of baking powder

For candied almonds

- around 10 almonds, roughly chopped

- 1 tablespoon of maple syrup or honey

- ½ teaspoon of ground cinnamon

Method

1. Preheat the oven to 350 degrees F (180 C).

2. Prepare 4 small-sized baking moulds with dairy-free butter and set aside.

3. In a large bowl, combine the almond milk with the coconut oil, carrot puree and sugar. Whisk using a blender.

4.   Slowly add the rice flour and fold it in using a spoon. Ensure there are no lumps in the mixture.

5.   Add the cocoa and baking powder. Mix again.

6.   Fill the muffin moulds about halfway up with this batter. Set aside.

7.   Place a piece of parchment paper on a flat microwave dish.

8.   Combine the almonds with the maple syrup and ground cinnamon and spread that mixture over the dish.

9.   Place the muffin moulds and the tray with the almonds in the oven and bake for 15 minutes.

10.   Remove the almonds and allow the cakes to bake for 10 more minutes.

11.   Take the cakes out of the moulds, top them with almond candies and serve.

4. Gluten Free Carrot Soufflé

Serves: 8

Ingredients

- 2 lbs carrots
- ¾ cup of sugar
- 1 ½ teaspoons of baking powder
- 1 ½ teaspoons of vanilla extract
- ½ teaspoon of cinnamon
- ¼ teaspoon of nutmeg
- ¼ teaspoon of ground black pepper
- 2 heaping tablespoons of gluten-free flour
- 3 egg-whites
- ½ cup of dairy-free butter, softened
- 2 tablespoons of grated carrot for topping
- 2 tablespoons of icing sugar for topping

Method

1. Preheat the oven to 350 degrees F (180 C).

2. Wash, peel and dice the carrots.

3. Fill a large pot with 2-3 cups of water. Bring the water to a boil and add the carrots to it.

4.   Cover the pot and cook the carrots until they are tender (about 5 minutes).

5.   Once they cool down, drain the excess water and add them to a blender.

6.   Add the sugar, baking powder, vanilla, cinnamon, nutmeg and pepper.

7.   Blend until a smooth paste is obtained and transfer to a bowl.

8.   Mix in the flour, eggs and softened dairy-free butter.

9.   Transfer to a prepared baking tray and bake for about an hour. You want the top to be golden brown.

10.   Top with icing sugar and grated carrots.

5. Low FODMAP Coconut Chiffon Spice Cake

Serves: 12

Ingredients

- 3 cups of all-purpose flour
- ½ teaspoon of baking soda
- 1 teaspoon of baking powder
- ½ teaspoon of salt
- ½ teaspoon of ground nutmeg
- 1 tablespoon of xanthan gum
- ¼ teaspoon of clove powder
- 2 cups of sugar
- 5 tablespoons of dairy-free butter
- 6 egg-whites and yolks
- 2 teaspoons of almond extract
- 2 teaspoons of vanilla extract
- 1 cup of virgin coconut oil
- 1 cup of coconut milk
- ¾ cup of desiccated coconut

Method

1. Preheat the oven to 350 degrees F (180 C).

2. Prepare a baking tray with cooking spray.

3. In a bowl, combine the all-purpose flour with the baking soda, baking powder, salt, nutmeg powder, xanthan gum and clove powder. Mix well.

4. In another bowl, combine the sugar with the dairy-free butter. Whisk using a blender until it becomes nice and fluffy.

5. Separate the egg yolks from the egg whites. Keep both.

6. Whisk the egg yolks with a blender until they are frothy.

7. Add almond extract, vanilla extract and coconut oil to the yolk mixture. Mix well.

8. Now use the blender to whisk the egg-whites until you see soft peaks.

9. Pour the yolk mixture into the flour mixture slowly while adding the coconut milk. Whisk slightly using the blender.

10. Gently fold the desiccated coconut and egg-whites into the batter.

11. Pour the batter into the prepared tin.

12. Bake for 45 to 50 minutes and allow it to cool on a rack for the 15 minutes.

13.   Slice and serve or store in an airtight container for up to 7 days.

6. FODMAP Free Sour Cream Ice Cream

Serves: 4

Ingredients

- 2 large cups of French vanilla creamer

- 2 tablespoons of coconut oil

- ¼ teaspoon of guar gum

- 1 tablespoon of vanilla extract

- 1 cup of granulated sugar

- 8 egg-whites and yolks

- 4 cups of sour cream (FODMAP free)

- 7-8 almonds, chopped

Method

1.   In a nonreactive bowl, combine the French vanilla creamer with the coconut oil, guar gum, vanilla extract and sugar. Whisk using a blender. Blend until slightly frothy condition. Do not over-whisk.

2.   Transfer this mixture to a large saucepan and bring it to a boil over medium heat. Remove it from the heat to cool.

3.   Using another nonreactive bowl, separate the egg whites from the yolks and only use the yolks. Whisk them until they are nice and frothy.

4.   Add the creamed mixture slowly to the egg yolk mixture, stirring continuously. Whisk it using a blender, a whisk or a large spoon.

5.   Add all of this back to the saucepan and heat it until it reaches 170 degrees F (80 C) on a thermometer. Remove from heat.

6.   Gently fold in the sour cream.

7.   Add the chopped almonds and pour everything into an ice cream mould.

8.   Refrigerate for about 6 hours and serve.

7. Low FODMAP Chocolate Peanut Butter Lava Cakes

Serves: 4

Ingredients

- five or six ramekins

- dairy-free butter and flour for coating and dusting ramekins

- 2-3 cups of water

- 7 tablespoons of dairy-free butter

- 1 ½ cup of bittersweet chocolate chips

- 3 tablespoons of peanut butter

- 1 tablespoons of confectionary sugar

- 1 tablespoon of dark cocoa powder

- 3 large egg-whites

- ¼ cup of gluten-free all-purpose flour

- 12-14 walnuts, chopped

Method

1. Preheat the oven to 425 degrees F (220 C).

2. Brush about 5 to 6 ramekins (a small dish for baking and serving an individual portion of food) with some dairy-free butter and then dust them with flour.

3. Bring 2 to 3 cups of water to a boil.

4. Place a nonreactive bowl on top of the pot of water. Add the dairy-free butter and the chocolate chips to the bowl. Stir until both ingredients are melted completely.

5. In another bowl, combine the peanut butter with the sugar, cocoa powder and egg-whites.

6. Add the chocolate and butter mixture to the peanut butter bowl and beat the mixture using a blender.

7. Gently fold in the gluten-free flour.

8. Pour the batter into the dusted ramekins and top them with chopped walnuts.

9. Set the ramekins in the oven and bake for 15 minutes.

10. Let them cool on a rack for about 5 more minutes.

11. Dump out the cakes and place them on a plate.

12. Dust them with more granulated sugar and serve.

Chapter 11: Low FODMAP Dinners

1. Salmon & Lemon Mini Fish Cakes

Serves: 4

Ingredients

- 2 large potatoes

- 2 tablespoons of olive oil

- 1 teaspoon of sea salt

- 1 teaspoon of ground pepper

- 1 teaspoon of dried parsley

- ½ teaspoon of dried oregano

- 3 tablespoons of lemon juice

- zest of one lemon (save some for garnish)

- 1 cup of salmon trimmings

- 1 egg-white

- corn flour

- oil for frying

- chopped coriander for garnish

Method

1.   Wash the potatoes thoroughly.

2.   Bring a large container of water to a boil. Add the potatoes and cover. Cook for about 7 minutes until they are tender. Once the potatoes cool down, peel off the skins and mash them well with your hands. Set aside in a large bowl.

3.   Add the olive oil, salt, pepper, parsley, oregano, lemon juice and lemon zest (save some zest for garnish) to the mashed potatoes. Mix well.

4.   Add the salmon trimmings and mix again.

5.   Crack an egg on top of this mixture and knead it into a soft dough.

6.   Using your hands, make 15-18 small rounds.

7.   Roll these cakes in corn flour.

8.   Add a few drops of oil to a pan and heat over medium heat.

9.   Fry the salmon cakes for 3-4 minutes on each side until they are slightly crisp.

10.   Garnish with chopped coriander and lemon zest and serve.

2. Spiced Quinoa with Almonds and Feta

Serves: 4

Ingredients

- 1 ½ cups of quinoa

- 1 tablespoon of olive oil

- ½ teaspoon of turmeric

- 1 teaspoon of minced ginger

- 10-12 almonds, chopped

- 1 teaspoon of salt

- ½ teaspoon of cayenne pepper

- 1 tablespoon of lemon juice

- ½ a green chilli, finely chopped

- 1 cup of vegetable stock

- 5 tablespoons of feta cheese, grated

- fresh coriander, chopped, for garnish

- handful of freshly plucked parsley, chopped, for garnish

Method

1. Rinse the quinoa under running water and drain the excess water. Soak it for about 30 minutes.

2. Chop the almonds using a sharp knife and slightly toast them on a pan over medium heat.

3. Heat olive oil in a pan over medium heat.

4. Add the turmeric and minced ginger. Sauté for a couple of minutes.

5. Throw in the chopped almonds and fry for two more minutes.

6. Slide in the soaked quinoa along with the salt, pepper, lemon juice and green chilli. Fry until the quinoa turns slightly brown.

7. Add the vegetable stock and simmer for 5-6 minutes.

8. Cover with a lid and cook for a few more minutes until the quinoa is fully cooked.

9. Remove the lid and stir in the feta cheese.

10. Cover again and allow the cheese to melt.

11. Garnish with chopped fresh coriander.

12. Serve warm.

3. Low FODMAP Pumpkin and Carrot Risotto

Serves: 4

Ingredients

- 2 large carrots
- 1 cup of Japanese pumpkin
- 1 teaspoon of salt
- 1 teaspoon of ground black pepper
- 1 tablespoon of olive oil
- ½ cup of leek or scallions, chopped
- 2 cups of baby spinach, drained and roughly chopped
- 2 tablespoons of lemon juice
- 4 ½ cups of vegetable stock
- 1 ½ cup of risotto rice
- 2 teaspoons of lemon zest
- 4 tablespoons of grated Parmesan cheese
- fresh coriander, chopped, for garnish

Method

1. Preheat the oven to 390 degrees F (200 C).

2.   Wash and peel the carrots and slice them into small chunks.

3.   Season the carrots and pumpkin with salt and pepper. Place them on a prepared baking tray.

4.   Bake for 20 minutes until they are slightly golden. Set aside.

5.   Heat the oil in a large saucepan over medium heat.

6.   Add the leek and spinach. Sauté for 2-3 minutes until they are tender.

7.   Add the baked carrots and pumpkin along with more salt and pepper and the lemon juice. Fry for a minute.

8.   Slowly pour the vegetable stock into the pan by continuously stirring.

9.   Slide in the risotto rice and sprinkle with lemon zest. Cover with the lid.

10.   Cook for 20 minutes and remove from heat.

11.   Stir in the grated cheese, garnish with chopped coriander and serve.

4. Green Chicken Curry

Serves: 4

Ingredients

- 6 chicken thighs
- 1 ½ teaspoon of salt, divided
- 1 teaspoon of ground black pepper, divided
- 1 stalk of lemon grass, chopped
- 2 tablespoons of grated ginger
- 1 teaspoon of coriander
- 1 teaspoon of roasted cumin
- 2 medium green chilies, slit
- 2 teaspoons of sugar
- 4 kaffir lime leaves, chopped
- 2 tablespoons of olive oil
- 2 teaspoons of fish sauce
- 1 tablespoon of lemon juice
- 4 small carrots, peeled and chopped
- 1 large green bell pepper, sliced
- 2 cups of coconut milk

- chopped coriander and zest of one lemon for garnish

Method

1. Wash the chicken thighs and pat dry with paper towels. Season with salt and pepper.

2. Heat some olive oil in a large saucepan and add the chicken thighs to it. Cook them for about 4 minutes on each side until they are browned. Set them aside in a bowl.

3. Put in a blender: lemon grass, ginger, coriander, cumin, green chilies, black pepper, sugar, kaffir leaves, olive oil, fish sauce and lemon juice. Blend until a smooth paste is obtained.

4. Heat a large pan over medium heat.

5. Add the paste to the pan and fry for 2-3 minutes, until all the spices start releasing their flavor.

6. Throw in the chopped carrots and green bell pepper. Sauté for a couple of minutes until they will be tender.

7. Slide in the chicken thighs along with more salt and pepper. Stir well.

8. Add the coconut milk and let the curry simmer on low heat for about 40 minutes.

9. Sprinkle lemon zest and chopped coriander for garnish. Serve hot.

5. Spaghetti Bolognese

Serves: 4

Ingredients

- 1 tablespoon of olive oil

- 2 cups of ground beef

- 2 cups of crushed tomatoes

- 3 cups of baby spinach, roughly chopped

- 1 medium carrot, peeled and sliced

- ½ cup of chopped leek or scallions

- 3 tablespoons of tomato paste

- 1 teaspoon of dried oregano

- 1 teaspoon of dried basil

- 1 teaspoon of salt

- 1 teaspoon of ground black pepper

- 1 cup of gluten-free spaghetti (1 package)

- ¼ cup of grated parmesan cheese for garnish

- chopped parsley for garnish

Method

1. Heat some oil in a large saucepan over medium heat.

2.   Add the ground beef and cook for 3 to 4 minutes until it turns brown.

3.   Add the crushed tomatoes to the cooked beef along with baby spinach, chopped carrot and leek. Mix well.

4.   Allow the mixture to simmer for a good 20 minutes, so the sauce thickens. Don't forget to keep stirring the mixture during its thickening, so it doesn't scorch.

5.   Add the tomato paste, dried oregano, basil, salt and pepper. Toss the ingredients well.

6.   In the meanwhile, bring about 3 cups of water to a boil in a large pot. Turn down the heat and add the spaghetti. Cook for about 10-12 minutes as per directions on the packet. Drain the excess water and quickly add some cold water to the spaghetti, so it doesn't stick together. Wait for 30 seconds and then drain the cold water too. Transfer the spaghetti to a large dish.

7.   Put the beef mixture on top of the spaghetti.

8.   Garnish with grated cheese and chopped parsley.

9.   Serve hot.

6. Quinoa Crusted Chicken Parmesan

Serves: 4 to 5

Ingredients

- 4 medium chicken breasts

- 1 teaspoon of salt, divided

- 1 teaspoon of ground black pepper, divided

- 3-4 cups of water

- 2 cups of quinoa

- 1 ½ cup of almond milk

- ½ cup of potato starch

- 2 egg-whites

- ¼ cup of parmesan cheese

- 1 cup of marinara sauce for topping

- fresh basil leaves, chopped, for garnish

Method

1.   Wash the chicken breasts and pat dry using paper towels. Season with salt and pepper.

2.   Heat a large pan and cook the chicken thighs for about 2 minutes on each side until they are slightly tender. Set aside.

3.   Add about 3-4 cups of water to a large pot and bring it to a boil.

4.   Slide in the quinoa and cook for about 5 minutes, covered. Drain the excess water, when it is done, transfer the quinoa to a large plate.

5.   Put some almond milk in a bowl and set aside.

6.   Add the potato starch along with some salt and pepper to another bowl and set aside.

7.   Crack the egg-whites into a small bowl and gently whisk them using a spoon.

8.   Prepare a baking tray with some cooking oil.

9.   Dip the chicken breasts in the almond milk and then into the potato starch mixture.

10.   Then dip them in the whisked egg-whites and finally coat them with the quinoa.

11.   Top each chicken breast with Parmesan cheese.

12.   Bake for 25 minutes and then cool.

13.   Add some marinara sauce on top and then sprinkle on chopped basil leaves for garnish.

14.   Serve hot.

7. Chili Coconut Crusted Fish with Homemade Chips & Salad

Serves: 3

Ingredients

For the crust

- ¼ cup of shredded coconut, dried

- 2 tablespoons of sesame oil

- 1 small mild green chilli, sliced

- ¼ cup of shallots, chopped

- 4-5 kaffir lime leaves, roughly chopped

- 2 cups of white flesh fish

- ¾ teaspoon of salt

- ½ teaspoon of ground black pepper

For the chips

- 4 medium potatoes, peeled and thinly sliced

- ½ teaspoon of salt

- ½ teaspoon of ground black pepper

- Spar cooking oil

For the salad

- 1 medium cucumber

- 4 cups lettuce, washed and sliced into strips

- 1 small red bell pepper, sliced into strips

- 1 tablespoon of lemon juice

- ¼ teaspoon of salt

- ¼ teaspoon of ground black pepper

Method

1.   Add the shredded coconut to a bowl of water. Soak it for 10-12 minutes and then drain the excess water.

2.   Heat the sesame oil in a large pan over medium heat.

3.   Add the sliced green chilli, chopped shallots and kaffir leaves to the pan. Fry until the leaves release their fragrance.

4.   Add the soaked coconut and fry for couple of minutes longer until it is slightly crisp.

5.   In the meantime, coat the sliced potatoes well with salt and pepper.

6.   Spray some cooking oil on another pan and heat over medium heat.

7.   Throw in the potato slices and fry them on both sides until they are brown and crisp. Move them to a large plate.

8.   In a bowl, combine all the ingredients for the salad and toss well.

9.   Heat a saucepan over low heat and add the fish to it. Fry for 2 minutes until it is slightly tender.

10.   Transfer the fish onto the same plate as the chips.

11.   Add the coconut chili filling on top and serve along with salad.

8. Tzatziki

Serves: 6

Ingredients

- 3 cups of dairy-free yoghurt

- juice of 1 lemon (about 3 tablespoons from a jar)

- 1 or 2 cloves garlic, chopped (garlic is okay here, because it is not cooked)

- 2 medium cumbers, peeled

- 1 tablespoon of salt (for salting the cucumbers to dry them out)

- 1 tablespoon of finely chopped fresh dill (or mint)

- salt and ground black pepper to taste

Method

1.   Peel the cucumbers, because insecticides or herbicides might be stored in the skin. If the cucumbers are organic, wash them and don't bother to peel them.

2.   Slice the cucumbers.

3.   Put the cucumber slices in a colander. Put salt on each slice. The salt is to draw the water out of them. You can layer the slices.

4.   Put them in the fridge or leave them on the counter. Give the salt at least 30 minutes to work. You can leave it for hours.

5.   Rinse the salt off the cucumber slices under running water. Dump the cucumber slices out on a clean towel and pat them dry. The drier — the better. We want cucumber taste and don't want cucumber water.

6.   Put the cucumber slices in a blender or food processor.

7.   Add the garlic, lemon juice, dill (or mint)and a generous grinding of black pepper. Whip it all into a smoothie.

8.   Put the dairy-free yogurt into a large bowl and dump the ingredients from the blender into that. Use a hand blender or a whisk to mix. You will see it turn from green to white.

9.   Taste and add some salt or pepper, if it is needed.

10.   Put a lid on the bowl and leave it in the fridge for at least two hours to let the flavours blend.

11.   Tzatziki is best used for souvlaki, but it is a spectacular dip for veggies, such as broccoli sprigs or carrot sticks. You can keep this in the fridge for a week.

9. Salad Dressing

Ingredients

- 1 cup of olive oil

- 1/3 cup of balsamic vinegar

- 2-3 tablespoons of red wine vinegar

- some salt to taste

Optional Ingredients

- Dijon mustard

- brown sugar

- shallots, minced (instead of garlic)

- ground black pepper

- lemon juice

- whatever else you can think of

Method

1. Combine balsamic vinegar with olive oil to your personal taste, more oil than vinegar. Add red wine vinegar for some bite. Then add a bit of salt.

2. Add other things, if you wish to. There are some suggestions above. Use your imagination. Just keep it on the low FODMAP.

3. Mix well and pour into a nice glass jar, maybe one that used to contain olive oil.

4.   If you added any fresh ingredients, such as minced shallots or lemon juice, you must keep this dressing in the fridge. If you don't include fresh ingredients, you can keep the jar on the counter and it will not go bad.

5.   Another thing to keep in mind is that you can whip this up at the drop of a hat. There are no rules. A splash of olive oil and a smaller splash of balsamic vinegar. Whisk or shake. Throw in some red wine vinegar, if you have it. This is the basic and it is yummy and much better for you than any commercial salad dressing. And it's different every time you make it, which is kind of fun.

We hope you enjoy our recipes and, if you don't cook, at least be cognizant of the things you should not eat. Happy times!

Made in United States
Troutdale, OR
12/14/2024

26422879R00060